Declutter Your Life for Peace and Purpose

A Practical Guide to Mindful Living and Simplified Spaces

Author

Yimam Beshir   Dec. 2024

Copyright

Dedication

To those seeking peace in a chaotic world. This book is for you.

Acknowledgments

I extend my heartfelt gratitude to my family for their unwavering support throughout this journey. To my spouse, who patiently endured late nights and countless revisions with unwavering encouragement, and to my children, whose boundless imagination served as a constant source of inspiration.

A special thanks to my mother, Yetemegn Asfaw, for her steadfast encouragement and tireless championing of this work. My appreciation also goes to the editorial review team at Amazon KDP for their insightful feedback, which significantly enriched this manuscript, and for providing a platform to bring this vision to life.

I am deeply thankful to Dr. Hassen Beshir for his invaluable insights and constructive criticism, which strengthened the narrative and refined the final work.

This book would not have been the same without the exceptional cover design and illustrations made possible through Canva's free plan, which brought my vision to life with creativity and vibrancy.

Finally, to you, the reader, thank you for embarking on this journey with me. Your imagination breathes life into these characters and gives this story its true home.

Preface

During my journey toward minimalism, I remember standing in my overflowing closet, overwhelmed by the sheer number of items I rarely wore. The moment I decided to let go of what no longer served me—donating dozens of pieces to those in need—I felt an incredible sense of relief and clarity. That decision marked the beginning of a lifestyle transformation, one where I chose simplicity and intentionality over excess. Sharing this story, I hope to inspire readers to reflect on their own spaces and take that first step toward meaningful decluttering.

Table of Content

Introduction

Why We Keep Buying More

In today's world, where consumerism often equates happiness with acquiring more, the philosophy of minimalism emerges as a countercultural yet deeply meaningful approach to life. Minimalism isn't about deprivation; instead, it's about intentionally choosing simplicity to focus on what truly matters. The art of living with less isn't about the number of items you own; it's about fostering a mindful relationship with your possessions and prioritizing quality, purpose, and gratitude. This chapter delves into the core principles of minimalism, guiding you to uncover your "enough," adopt a quality-over-quantity mindset, and embrace gratitude as a transformative practice for intentional living.

Defining Your "Enough"

Minimalism begins with understanding what "enough" means for you personally. This process is deeply introspective—a journey of differentiating your true needs from your wants. For instance, recognizing that owning a reliable car to commute might be a need, while yearning for the latest sports car might be a want. It's about stripping away external pressures, such as societal expectations to own more or achieve a certain status, to uncover the essentials that align with your values and lifestyle.

How to Define Your Enough

Ask Reflective Questions: Start by asking yourself: Which items do I truly need to feel comfortable and functional in my daily life? What possessions bring genuine joy or add meaningful value to my existence? Which things could I release without a sense of loss?

Focus on Function and Purpose: Pinpoint what enables you to live contentedly without excess. Evaluate whether an item serves its purpose well or simply takes up space.

Personalizing Your Minimalism

Your definition of enough is entirely unique. By answering these questions, you create a framework for making decisions about which belongings to retain and which to let go. Start by listing your essential needs and values, then sort your belongings into categories—essential, meaningful, and unnecessary. This clarity allows you to build a lifestyle truly aligned with your needs—free of unnecessary clutter but enriched with meaningful possessions.

Creating an Inventory of Essentials

Once you understand your definition of "enough," the next step is to assess your current belongings and create a personal inventory. This practice not only declutters your life but also reinforces a conscious simplicity by categorizing your possessions.

Steps to Build Your Inventory:

List Your Essentials: Identify the items you rely on daily or weekly. These might include pieces of clothing, kitchen tools, or gadgets. Highlight their importance and usefulness in your routine.

Evaluate Sentimental Items: Recognize belongings tied to memories. Keep only those that evoke joy or hold significant meaning to your personal story. Let go of items lying idle that no longer resonate.

Identify What Can Be Released: Dive into the cornered clutter—possessions collecting dust.

Decide whether to donate, recycle, or discard these items with thoughtfulness.

Benefits of a Personal Inventory

This reflective inventory process helps streamline your environment, ensuring that everything remaining has a purpose or value. Over time, this practice reduces the emotional and mental weight of excess, leaving you with a space that breathes simplicity and intent.

The Value of Quality Over Quantity

A cornerstone of minimalism is shifting focus from amassing numerous possessions to choosing high-quality, versatile ones. This approach not only reduces clutter but also ensures that every item serves a meaningful purpose.

How to Prioritize Quality

Durability First: Opt for items made from materials designed to last—sturdy clothing, reliable kitchen tools, or long-lasting furniture. High-quality products reduce the need for frequent replacements, saving resources and reducing waste.

Versatility Matters: Select multipurpose items wherever possible. For example, a cast iron skillet can be used for various cooking techniques, while modular furniture adapts to changing needs.

Mindful Purchasing: Before any purchase, ask yourself: Will this item genuinely enhance my life? Does it align with the lifestyle I'm curating? This question helps avoid impulsive buying and ensures new additions hold significance.

Benefits of Choosing Quality

Focusing on quality drives conscious consumption and promotes long-term satisfaction. Your living spaces become more streamlined, functional, and aesthetically pleasing, reinforcing the essence of a life lived with intention.

Cultivating a Gratitude Practice

Gratitude is a transformative component of minimalism. By appreciating what you already have, the desire for excess diminishes, leaving space for contentment and simplicity to thrive.

Techniques to Foster Gratitude:

Daily Reflections: Spend just a few minutes each day reflecting on the things you're grateful for. It could be simple pleasures like a warm cup of tea, a favorite book, or the support of loved ones.

Gratitude Journaling: Maintain a journal and write down three things you appreciate each day. This consistent practice helps center your attention on abundance rather than what's missing.

Mindful Consumption: Before purchasing something new, pause and ask, "Do I truly need this? Will it add value to my life?" Reflecting on these questions encourages thoughtful choices.

Expressing Appreciation: Share your gratitude with others. A simple "thank you" or an act of kindness can deepen relationships and promote a culture of appreciation.

Why Gratitude Matters

Gratitude shifts focus from lack to abundance, transforming how you view your life and possessions. As part of your minimalist journey, it fosters a sense of fulfillment, making the pursuit of more feel unnecessary while enhancing the joy found in what you already have.

Conclusion

Minimalism is not just about owning fewer things; it's a lifestyle of embracing what truly matters. By defining your "enough," creating an inventory of essentials, focusing on quality over quantity, and practicing gratitude, you can transform your life in meaningful ways. Start your journey today and discover the freedom, clarity, and joy that come with living intentionally.

Each step you take toward minimalism creates space—both physical and mental—for what brings you joy and fulfillment. The weight of unnecessary possessions lifts, making room for freedom, clarity, and enriched living. Through this intentional approach, you'll discover the profound beauty of simplicity—where having less allows you to experience more.

As you embark on this journey, remember that minimalism is deeply personal. It's not a rigid set of rules but a path to curating a life that aligns with your values. Embrace the liberation, the calm, and the sense of purpose that comes with living intentionally.

In modern society, clutter has become a natural byproduct of a culture driven by consumerism. The allure of advertisements, coupled with the convenience of instant purchases, creates an environment where the accumulation of material goods feels almost inevitable. Consumer culture often promises happiness and success through acquiring more, but in truth, this cycle frequently leads to stress, dissatisfaction, and an unfulfilling pursuit of "enough."

Consumerism fosters an insidious cycle: buy, use briefly, discard, and repeat. While the initial thrill of obtaining something new can be gratifying, it's often fleeting. Over time, this lifestyle promotes unproductivity and dissatisfaction, as the accumulation of material possessions fails to deliver lasting contentment. Studies indicate that constant consumerism amplifies stress, diminishes focus, and diverts our attention from the experiences and relationships that truly matter. In the process, we compromise mental well-being for clutter and excess.

Now imagine a life unburdened by the need to constantly acquire more. Picture a serene, uncluttered home where every belonging hold meaning and purpose. This kind of space fosters clarity and creativity, empowering you to focus on the experiences and relationships that matter most. Beyond the physical, this freedom extends to mental clarity and emotional peace—a life filled with less noise and more substance. By releasing ourselves from the grips of overconsumption, we can rediscover what it means to truly live and thrive.

Decluttering goes far deeper than organizing—it's the first step in reshaping the way we approach life. It challenges the mindset that acquiring more will lead to happiness while encouraging intentionality in every choice we make. By shifting this perspective, we can break free from the consumer trap, redefine what truly matters, and create room for joy, peace, and meaningful connections. Decluttering becomes an act of liberation, a way to reclaim our time, energy, and mental freedom from the overwhelming pressures of consumer culture.

Chapter1.Understanding Consumerism

1.1. Modern Spending Habits

What is Consumerism?

Consumerism can be broadly defined as a social and economic framework that encourages the acquisition of goods and services in increasing amounts. At its core, consumerism reflects the idea that personal well-being and happiness heavily depend on levels of consumption and material possessions. This concept has evolved over centuries, underpinned by developments in advertising, industrialization, and global trade.

The History of Consumer Culture

"The roots of consumer culture trace back to industrialization in the 18th and 19th centuries (Kasser, 2002)", when mass production made goods more accessible to the general public. As manufacturing efficiency grew, so did the need for businesses to create demand. Enter advertising— crafted to appeal to human desires, aspirations, and insecurities. From the rise of department stores to modern online shopping platforms, consumer culture has only intensified over the decades.

1.2. How Advertising Shapes Our Desires

"Modern advertising employs psychological strategies to influence our decision-making (Smith, 2019)." Techniques such as emotional appeals, the use of aspirational imagery, and even the deliberate creation of scarcity manipulate us into associating consumption with fulfillment and success. Think of how ads equate owning the latest gadget or designer product with prestige and identity. This constant bombardment reinforces a cycle where consumers feel the need to buy more and new items to stay relevant or satisfied.

1.3. The Psychological Tricks Behind Modern Marketing

From leveraging FOMO (Fear of Missing Out) to exploiting our cognitive biases, marketing today is more sophisticated and pervasive than ever before. Subtle strategies like the use of social proof (e.g.,

"Everyone is buying this!") or targeted personalization through data mining make advertisements feel irresistible. This unrelenting exposure often results in impulsive buying habits, blurring the line between need and want.

Why Do We Fall into the Trap?

The allure of consumerism isn't a coincidence; it's a psychological and social phenomenon, carefully engineered to tap into our emotions and social instincts.

Emotional Spending: Buying Happiness or Status

Emotional spending often stems from the belief that material possessions will bring happiness or elevate social standing. People frequently shop as a way to cope with stress, boredom, or sadness—a phenomenon known as retail therapy. While buying provides a temporary sense of satisfaction, it seldom leads to long-term happiness. Instead, it can create a cycle of emotional dependency on material goods to fill emotional voids.

In addition, many purchases are driven not by utility but by the desire to signal status. Luxury items, for instance, are often marketed as symbols of success and opulence, encouraging consumers to equate their value with their possessions. This can lead to a pursuit of fleeting validation rather than genuine contentment.

1.4.   The Role of Social Media in Fueling FOMO

Social media platforms amplify consumerism through constant exposure to curated lifestyles and possessions. The "highlight reels" of influencers and friends showcase exotic vacations, fancy gadgets, and trendy outfits, fueling feelings of inadequacy and FOMO (Fear of Missing Out). Platforms use algorithms to ensure users are continually exposed to this content, often paired seamlessly with advertisements, further entrenching the idea that consumption is central to belonging and happiness.

Moreover, social media incentivizes behaviors like brand loyalty and impulse buying through flash sales, influencers' discount codes, and "buy now" features. It's a digital-age playground for psychological triggers that drive people directly to virtual shopping carts.

1.5.　　The Hidden Costs of Buying More

While consumerism offers the allure of new and shiny possessions, the hidden costs tied to excessive consumption can have far-reaching impacts beyond what meets the eye.

Financial Strain

Overindulgence in consumerism often leads to financial instability. Credit card debt, impulsive purchases, and the pressure to keep up with others' lifestyles can cause serious financial burdens. Instead of saving or investing, many individuals end up living paycheck-to-paycheck, creating long-term economic fragility.

Environmental Harm

The environmental footprint of consumerism is enormous. From the depletion of natural resources to the overflowing landfills and pollution caused by waste, growing consumer demand takes a significant toll on the planet. Fast fashion is a prime example, with cheaply produced yet short-lived garments creating unsustainable waste streams.

Moreover, the energy-intensive production pipelines contribute to greenhouse gas emissions, exacerbating global climate change.

Emotional Tolls

Ironically, while consumerism promises happiness, it often yields the opposite. The constant pursuit of more can lead to feelings of dissatisfaction, stress, and anxiety. People may tie their self-worth to external possessions, creating an identity crisis when financial or material circumstances change. Furthermore, the clutter from excessive possessions often overwhelms, reducing one's mental well-being rather than enhancing it.

1.6. Understanding Mindful and Emotional Spending

How people spend their money has a big impact on their financial health and well-being. Mindful spending means making thoughtful purchases that align with one's values and goals, while emotional spending refers to buying driven by impulses or feelings without considering long-term effects.

Mindful Spending

Mindful spending is characterized by its purpose-driven nature. It fulfills immediate or long-term needs and aligns closely with an individual's financial objectives and lifestyle. Purchases made under this umbrella tend to be planned and deliberate. For instance, essential expenditures like grocery items, gym memberships, and medications serve fundamental needs such as sustenance and well-being, while work-related expenses such as professional tools are necessary for career advancement. Such spending reflects a conscientious approach to financial decision-making, wherein each purchase is considered for its utility and relevance to personal values.

Emotional Spending

In contrast, emotional spending is often cluttered and unnecessary, driven primarily by impulses rather than genuine needs. This type of spending is frequently triggered by emotions such as stress or boredom, as well as external pressures like social influence. Unlike mindful purchases, emotional spending only provides temporary satisfaction and misaligns with long-term financial goals. Examples include buying items on sale that one doesn't truly need or acquiring gadgets due to fear of missing out. Such decisions often lead to regret and financial strain, as they add clutter without lasting value.

SHOPPING HABIT TRACK

Category	Total Spending ($)	Reflection
Mindful Purchases	$___	How did these purchases add value?
Emotional Purchases	$___	What could you avoid in the future?
Net Savings/Loss	$___	What did you save by avoiding clutter?

Net saving or loss after spending habits

Table 1. Net saving or loss after spending habits

1.7.   How to Decide Cluttered and Decluttered Spending

Making thoughtful spending decisions can help you differentiate between cluttered and decluttered purchases, ensuring your financial choices align with your broader goals. By evaluating purchases through reflective questions, alternatives, and impact assessments, you can develop a more intentional approach to spending.

Ask Reflective Questions

Before making a purchase, pause and ask yourself the following: Taking a moment to reflect helps you assess whether the purchase aligns with your needs, values, or goals. This mindful approach can prevent impulsive decisions and lead to more thoughtful, meaningful choices.

- Does this purchase serve a genuine need?

- Will it bring lasting value or solve a problem in my life?
- Could I wait 24 hours to make this purchase?

These simple yet powerful questions disrupt impulse-driven decisions and encourage you to think critically about whether the purchase supports your needs and goals. For example, asking, "Will I still value this item in a month?" or "Does this align with what I truly need right now?" can help you pause and reconsider. Patience and reflection often reveal purchases that would otherwise add clutter without meaningful benefit.

Consider Alternatives

Sometimes, the solution you're seeking doesn't even require a new purchase. Considering alternatives not only saves money but also supports environmental sustainability by reducing waste and unnecessary consumption. For example:

- Instead of buying another coffee mug, could you declutter your current collection and appreciate what you already own?
- Would borrowing, reusing, or even DIYing fulfill the same purpose effectively?

These alternatives not only save money but also instill a sense of resourcefulness and appreciation for the items you already possess.

Impact Assessment

Finally, evaluate how the purchase contributes to your life:

- Decluttered Purchase: Adds value, reduces stress, and aligns with your personal and financial goals.
- Cluttered Purchase: Adds to physical, financial, or emotional clutter without addressing a genuine need or improving your quality of life.

By thoughtfully distinguishing between items that enrich your life and those that burden it, you create space—both literally and metaphorically—for what truly matters. Embrace this intentional mindset to foster lasting financial wellness and a clutter-free lifestyle.

In summary, recognizing the essential differences between mindful and emotional spending can empower individuals to make informed financial choices. By emphasizing the importance of purpose-driven purchases that align with personal values, one can cultivate a more sustainable and fulfilling financial future. In contrast, identifying and minimizing the impact of emotional spending can help reduce unnecessary financial burdens, ultimately leading to a more disciplined and intentional approach to expenditure. To put these insights into practice, start by tracking spending habits to identify patterns of emotional spending. Set clear financial goals that reflect personal values, and create a monthly budget to prioritize intentional purchases. Additionally, practicing mindfulness techniques, such as pausing before making a purchase or assessing whether it aligns with long-term objectives, can further support mindful spending strategies.

Chapter 2: Identifying Your Triggers

Understanding Emotional and External Triggers

Emotional Triggers in Consumer Spending

Emotions significantly influence consumer behavior, often driving impulsive spending. Stress can lead to impulsive purchases as individuals seek temporary relief or comfort. Similarly, boredom motivates shopping as a form of entertainment or distraction. Insecurity often causes individuals to spend on items aimed at boosting self-esteem or gaining social acceptance. Identifying these triggers allows for improved self-awareness and more mindful spending.

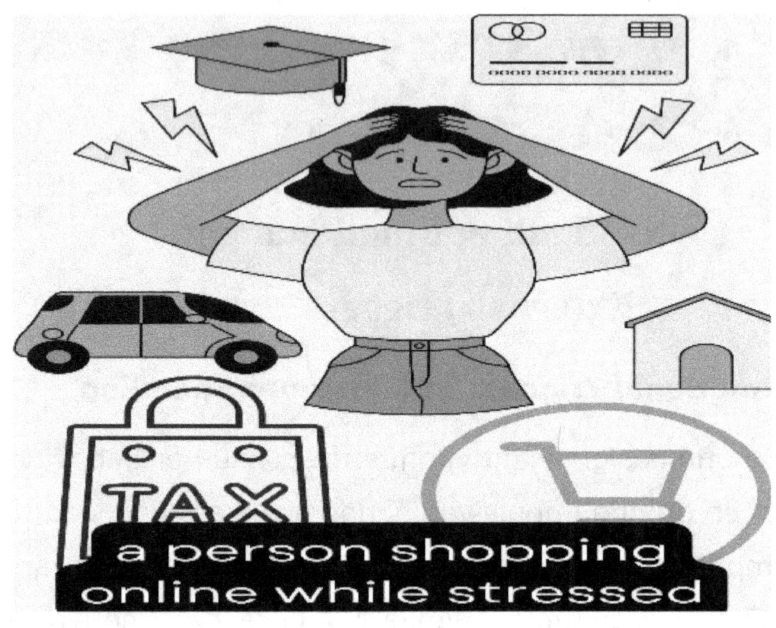

Figure 1: Shopper reactions to impulsive spending habits leads to stress illustrating how these tactics influence consumer decisions and the balance between wants and needs.

External Triggers in Consumer Behavior

External triggers are key factors in influencing purchasing decisions. Advertisements often exploit psychological tactics such as urgency and exclusivity, creating a fear of missing out (FOMO). Limited-time offers and seasonal sales events drive immediate action from consumers. Additionally, social media influencers play a considerable role, with their endorsements and aspirational lifestyles prompting followers to emulate their purchases. By becoming conscious of these triggers, consumers can resist undue influence and exercise better purchasing discipline.

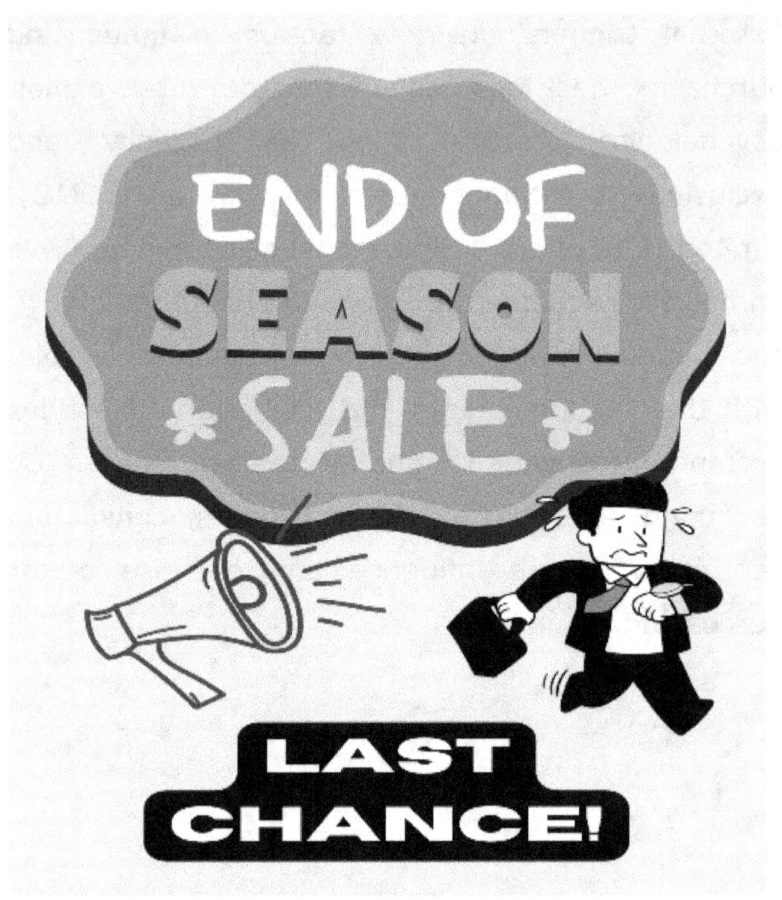

Figure 2: Why do we buy more than we need? This infographic explores how phrases like "Last Chance!" and "end of season sale" create urgency and shape our buying habits.

Journaling Exercise for Spending Awareness

Keeping a dedicated spending journal is an effective method for identifying emotional and external triggers. Individuals can record every purchase they make for a week, along with the feelings or reasons motivating each transaction. Analyzing this data reveals patterns, such as purchases driven by emotional responses or external pressures. This reflective process fosters awareness and helps in making more intentional financial decisions.

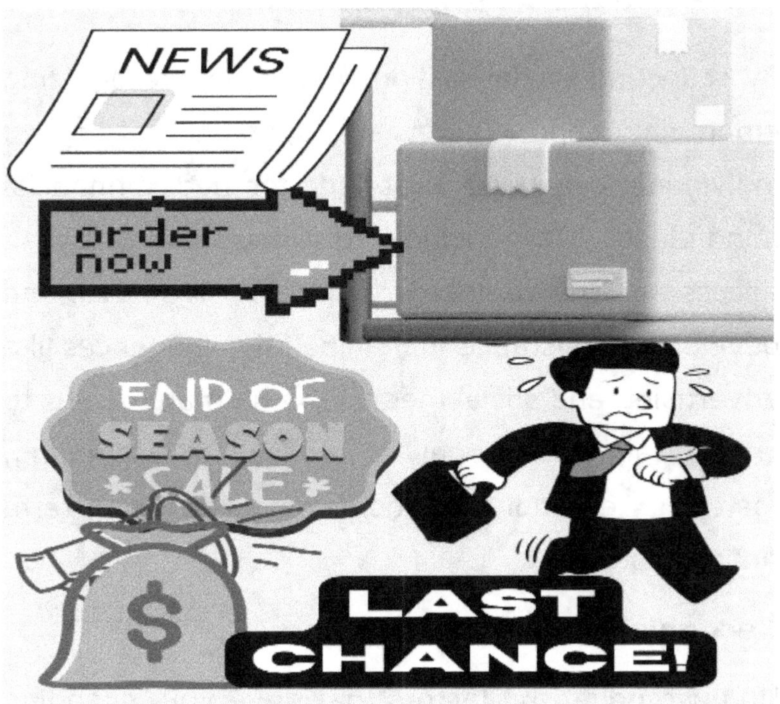

Figure 3: From " End of Season Sale" to "Last Chance" see how common marketing strategies impact the way we decide between wants and needs.

Achieving Financial Wellbeing

By reflecting on journaling results and recognizing emotional and external spending triggers, individuals can build strategies for better financial mindfulness. This includes distinguishing between necessities and wants, curbing impulsive buys, and developing resistance to manipulative influences like advertising and social media. The ultimate goal is to create an intentional approach to spending, fostering emotional satisfaction and long-term financial stability.

Recognizing Personal Triggers

Understanding the factors that drive your spending habits is a crucial step toward financial mindfulness. Triggers, whether emotional or external, can subtly influence your purchasing decisions, often without you even realizing it. Let's dive into these two primary types of triggers to gain a clearer understanding.

Emotional Triggers

Emotions are deeply tied to consumer behavior. Stress, for example, may lead to impulsive purchases as a way to seek temporary relief or comfort. You might find yourself clicking "Add to Cart" after a tiring day at work, hoping the new item will lift your spirits. Similarly, boredom can drive people to browse online stores or malls purely for entertainment, resulting in unnecessary purchases. Insecurity, on the other hand, might push individuals to spend on items designed to boost their self-esteem or help them gain social acceptance. Recognizing these patterns allows you to confront them and make more informed spending choices.

External Triggers

External triggers come from outside sources that aim to influence your buying decisions. Advertising is one of the strongest external triggers, masterfully employing tactics like urgency, exclusivity, and creating a fear of missing out (FOMO). For instance, phrases like "Buy Now! Limited Stock Available" can push you to act without thoroughly evaluating the purchase. Seasonal sales and promotional events, such as Black Friday or holiday discounts, capitalize on these principles. Additionally, social media influencers play a significant role; their endorsements and aspirational lifestyles often ignite the desire to emulate their choices.

By becoming aware of these external forces, you can build resilience and avoid making impulsive decisions based on persuasive marketing or peer influence.

Journaling Exercise

One of the most effective strategies to identify your spending triggers is through journaling. By keeping a spending journal for a week, you can gain incredible insights into your financial behaviors.

How to Log Your Spending

Record Every Purchase: Write down every single expense made during the week, no matter how small.

Reflect on Triggers: For each entry, note the emotion, situation, or external factor that influenced your decision to spend. Was it stress, boredom, or an advertisement?

Identify Patterns

At the end of the week, review your journal to spot recurring themes. Are there specific emotions or situations that consistently lead to purchases? Did certain types of ads or social media posts make you want to buy certain items? Answering these questions will help you better understand your personal spending drivers and take steps to manage or eliminate these triggers moving forward.

Chapter 3: Breaking Free from the Grip of Overconsumption

Overconsumption is one of the most significant contributors to clutter, stress, and financial strain in modern life. This chapter provides actionable strategies to help you break the cycle of unnecessary spending, regain control of your habits, and adopt a more intentional approach to consumption. By shifting your mindset and cultivating mindful shopping habits, you can pave the way for a clutter-free and purposeful life.

The "Pause and Reflect" Rule: Stop Impulsive Spending in Its Tracks

Before making any non-essential purchase, pause for 24-48 hours. This simple delay creates a buffer to reflect on whether the item is truly necessary or merely a result of emotional triggers or marketing tactics.

- **Why It Works:**

  1. Helps prevent impulsive decisions.

2. Allows you to differentiate between a genuine need and a fleeting desire.

- **How to Apply:**

1. Place the item on hold or leave it in your online shopping cart.

2. During this waiting period, ask yourself:

    - *Do I truly need this, or is it a momentary craving?*

    - *Will this item bring lasting value or joy to my life?*

    - *Can I borrow, reuse, or find a more sustainable alternative?*

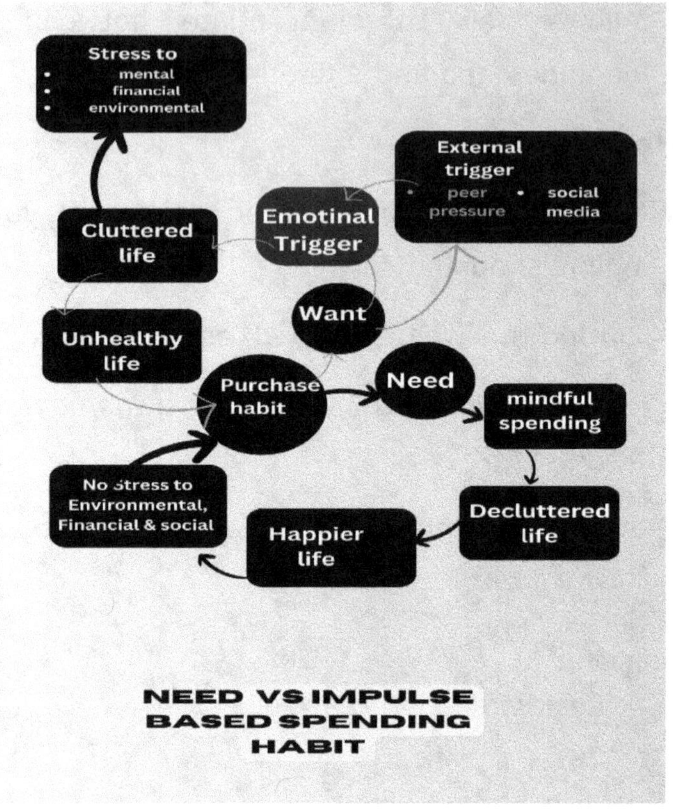

Figure 4. Showing the cycle of need and impulse purchase habit

Key Questions to Ask Yourself Before Buying

To further refine your decision-making process, consider these reflective questions. These can serve as a reminder checklist or even be written down in a spending mantra journal:

1. Do I really need this item, or can I make do without it?

2. Does this align with my long-term goals, values, or lifestyle?

3. Will this purchase genuinely enhance my well-being or happiness?

4. Am I buying this because of emotional triggers (stress, boredom, etc.)?

5. What would happen if I didn't buy this item right now?

These questions act as a litmus test, filtering out unnecessary purchases and encouraging intentional consumption.

Practice Mindful Shopping: Shop with Intention, Not Emotion

Mindful shopping is all about being deliberate and thoughtful when you engage in retail activities. By shopping with a clear purpose, you can avoid the common traps of consumerism and focus on fulfilling your genuine needs.

- **Tips for Practicing Mindful Shopping:**

  o Always create a shopping list and stick to it.

  o Set a monthly spending limit for non-essentials.

  o Avoid shopping as a form of entertainment or stress relief.

  o Beware of marketing traps, such as:

  a. "Limited-time offers" that pressure you into hurried decisions.

  b. "Buy one, get one free" deals that encourage overbuying.

- **The Power of Purposeful Shopping:**

  o Each purchase should align with your personal goals and values.

  o When you shop intentionally, you bring home items that truly matter.

Declutter First, Buy Later: Create Space Before Adding More

Before acquiring new possessions, make a habit of decluttering what you already own. This practice not only prevents your space from becoming overwhelmed but also fosters a mindset of appreciation for what you have.

- **Steps to Declutter Before Buying:**

1.   Take Inventory: Identify what you already have and assess its condition and usefulness.

2.   Eliminate Duplicates: If you find multiple items serving the same purpose, keep the best and donate or recycle the rest.

3.   Make Space: By clearing out old or unused items, you'll appreciate your space more and reduce the desire to fill it with new things.

- **The Decluttering Mantra:**

"Clear out the old to make space for the new—but only when the new adds value."

Bringing It All Together: A Sustainable Approach to Consumption

Breaking the cycle of overconsumption is not about deprivation—it's about empowerment. When you pause, reflect, and declutter, you create an environment that fosters peace, productivity, and purpose. You'll begin to see that a clutter-free life is not just about having less but about living more intentionally and meaningfully.

Chapter4. Power of Decluttering

Strategies and Practices for a Calm Life

In an increasingly cluttered world, the act of decluttering transcends mere tidiness; it signifies a profound mindset shift. "Decluttering reduces cortisol levels, the stress hormone, fostering a serene atmosphere (Chatzky, 2019)." It goes beyond simply letting go of possessions. Instead, it focuses on the myriad benefits that arise from creating physical and mental space. For instance, letting go of unnecessary items leads to a clearer mind, as there's less visual and mental noise. A clear mind is a focused state of mind that allows you to perform tasks without clouded thinking. It can be achieved by reducing an unwanted flow of thoughts and images, and simplifying your mental processes. By focusing on gains like tranquility and freedom instead of losses, individuals can foster a more enriching and harmonious living environment. Decluttering is thus not just cleaning but a deliberate and personal journey towards alignment with one's values and aspirations.

Decluttering as a Mindset Shift

For many, decluttering might seem daunting because it is immediately associated with loss. However, shifting the focus to what is gained—space, peace, and freedom—introduces a sense of purpose into the process. Imagine a home overwhelmed with forgotten objects, stifling physical and emotional space. Decluttering transforms such spaces into sanctuaries, enabling clearer thoughts and a calmer spirit. A clutter-free environment can enhance productivity, reduce stress, and even promote better sleep habits. It becomes essential to frame decluttering not as a loss but as a strategic reorganization that allows individuals to reclaim more control over their spaces and their lives. By embracing this mindset, decluttering transitions from being a chore to an empowering lifestyle choice.

Exploring Decluttering Methodologies

Several effective methodologies have emerged to support this journey, providing structure while encouraging flexibility. These methodologies make the daunting task of decluttering approachable and even enjoyable.

The KonMari Method: Sparking Joy

Perhaps the most renowned and transformative methodology is the KonMari Method, popularized by Marie Kondo. This approach posits a simple yet powerful question: "Does it spark joy? (Kondo, 2014). By holding each item and assessing its emotional resonance, individuals learn to differentiate between what truly matters and what does not. For instance, sentimental items such as old letters or family heirlooms can evoke hesitation. To resolve such hesitation, one might consider asking additional questions like "Does this item help me remember a cherished experience?" or "Can I preserve this memory in another meaningful way, such as a photograph?" The KonMari philosophy teaches us to honor these objects for the role they played in our lives but also to let go of those that no longer serve us or evoke happiness. This method encourages thoughtfulness, such as pausing to reflect on the purpose of each item; mindfulness, by being fully present in the act of decluttering and cherishing what we choose to keep; and intentionality, which involves making deliberate choices to create a living environment that aligns deeply with our personal values.

The Minimalist Game: Building Momentum Over Time

Another practical yet dynamic approach is the Minimalist Game. This technique gamifies the decluttering process, transforming it into a month-long challenge. Participants begin by letting go of one item on the first day, two on the second, three on the third, and so on, increasing the count incrementally over time. By the end of 30 days, approximately 465 items will have been removed. More than just a numerical exercise, this method fosters discipline and helps individuals build momentum. Highlighting daily progress, it instills a sense of achievement and demonstrates just how much can be gained when we commit to reducing excess baggage in our lives.

Decluttering Decision-Making Checklist

In an era characterized by consumerism and abundant possessions, the need for thoughtful decluttering has become increasingly significant due to its positive impact on mental health and its role in addressing environmental concerns. Thoughtful decluttering involves intentionally evaluating belongings, prioritizing those that add meaning or utility, and responsibly discarding or donating items that no longer serve a purpose. A structured approach to decluttering can facilitate decision-making, allowing individuals to cultivate a living space that reflects their values and needs. The following checklist serves as a guide to help assess items for retention or disposal, ensuring that each decision is made with intention and mindfulness.

Step 1: Evaluate the Item's Purpose

Begin by examining the practical utility of the item in question. Ask yourself whether it has a clear function in your daily life. It may no longer serve a meaningful purpose if the item has not been utilized in the past six months to a year— a range that typically allows enough time to factor in seasonal or occasional use. Furthermore, consider whether you anticipate using it soon; for instance, keeping an old gadget "just in case" or holding onto clothing that no longer fits while hoping it might fall into these "maybe someday" scenarios. In such cases, it may be prudent to reassess its place in your home to maintain a clutter-free environment.

Step 2: Assess Sentimental Value

Sentimental attachments can complicate the decluttering process. It is essential to differentiate between items that evoke genuine joy—those that bring a deep sense of happiness, fond memories, or personal meaning—and those retained out of guilt. For example, an old letter from a loved one that reminds you of treasured experiences might evoke joy, while an unused gift kept solely out of obligation might stem from guilt. If an item holds significant emotional value, it may warrant keeping. However, if guilt is the primary motivator for retention, it is advisable to release such feelings. Consider alternative methods of honoring memories, such as photographing the item to preserve its image or writing down its history and what it means to you. These approaches can help create a meaningful and less burdensome keepsake than the physical item itself.

Step 3: Check the Condition

The physical condition of an item is a crucial factor in the decision-making process. Items broken, damaged, or excessively worn may no longer justify retention. If an item has languished in a "to-repair" pile for an extended period, it may be time to let it go.

Step 4: Think About Space and Functionality

Evaluate the impact of the item on your living environment. Does it contribute to a sense of calm and organization, or does it add to the clutter? Consider whether you would prefer the space occupied by the item to remain empty. The act of freeing up space can be as rewarding as the act of holding onto possessions.

Step 5: Replaceability

Consider the replaceability of the item. If you did not already own it, would you choose to purchase it? If the answer is no, this may indicate that the item is not essential. Additionally, for items that are easily replaceable at low cost—such as under $20—or without significant emotional attachment, it may be wise to part with them. Reflecting on both the monetary and sentimental value of an item can make this decision more actionable.

Step 6: Consider Sharing or Donating

Lastly, reflect on the potential for the item to benefit others. If someone else could utilize the item more effectively than you, consider donating or gifting it. If the item holds considerable value and is in good condition, selling it may also be a viable option.

Mindful Shopping Reminder Checklist

To complement the decluttering process, a mindful shopping checklist can enhance intentional purchasing decisions.

Step 1: Need or Want?

Begin by distinguishing between needs and wants. Needs are essential, while wants may stem from impulse. Allowing a 24–48 hour pause before making a purchase can aid in assessing the item's true value.

Step 2: Usage and Functionality

Assess how often the item will be used. If it is not something you will utilize regularly, reconsider the purchase. Additionally, avoid acquiring duplicates unless absolutely necessary.

Step 3: Quality Over Quantity

Prioritize quality over quantity. Investing in durable items that align with your lifestyle can save money and reduce waste. Ensure that any potential purchase complements your existing wardrobe or home.

Step 4: Budget and Value

Evaluate whether the item is worth its price and consider its impact on your financial well-being. Avoid purchases that could lead to financial strain.

Step 5: Space and Storage

Before buying, ensure you have a designated space for the item. If no clear storage solution exists, it may contribute to clutter rather than enhance your environment.

Step 6: Environmental and Social Impact

Finally, consider the ethical implications of your purchase. Opt for environmentally friendly items that carry certifications like Fair Trade, USDA Organic, or Energy Star, and prioritize products made with sustainable materials or ethical labor practices. Think about the item's lifecycle, including whether it can be reused, repurposed as new items, or easily recycled at the end of its usefulness.

By utilizing these checklists, individuals can engage in more intentional decluttering and shopping practices.

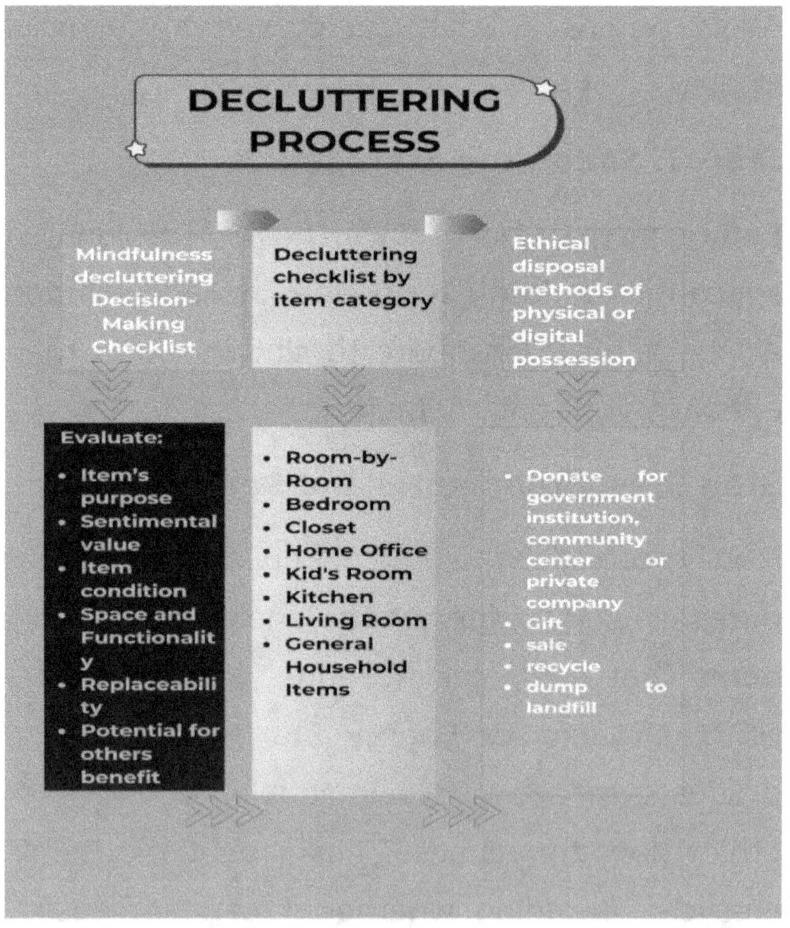

Figure 5. Showing Guidance on decluttering process

Room-by-Room Decluttering Checklist: Tackling Spaces Strategically

For those accustomed to visualizing progress and working systematically, a room-by-room decluttering checklist proves invaluable. This method involves breaking down the overwhelming task of decluttering into smaller, manageable projects. By choosing one space at a time—say the kitchen one week and the bedroom the next—the process can be made less intimidating. Additionally, lists help identify specific problem areas (e.g., a perpetually messy wardrobe) and ensure no part of a home is overlooked. Focused attention and regular reflection during this process allow individuals to think critically about what they truly require in each aspect of their lives.

What to Do with the Stuff: Ethical and Community-Oriented Disposals

A common challenge during decluttering is deciding what to do with items that no longer serve a purpose. Responsible disposal is crucial to the process. Items still in good condition can be donated to charitable organizations, sold in resale platforms, or gifted to individuals who may find value in them. For instance, donating clothes to a local shelter could provide much-needed warmth to someone in need. Similarly, recycling old electronic devices or paper materials can contribute positively to environmental sustainability. Responsible decluttering ensures that unwanted items are given new life rather than being relegated to landfills, aligning with both environmental and community-oriented ethical principles.

Resources for ethical disposal—such as local government recycling centers or community bulletin boards—are invaluable in finding homes for discarded possessions. On the digital front, platforms like eBay, Facebook Marketplace, and donation directories make it easier than ever to ensure that decluttering benefits not just the individual but also the community and the environment.

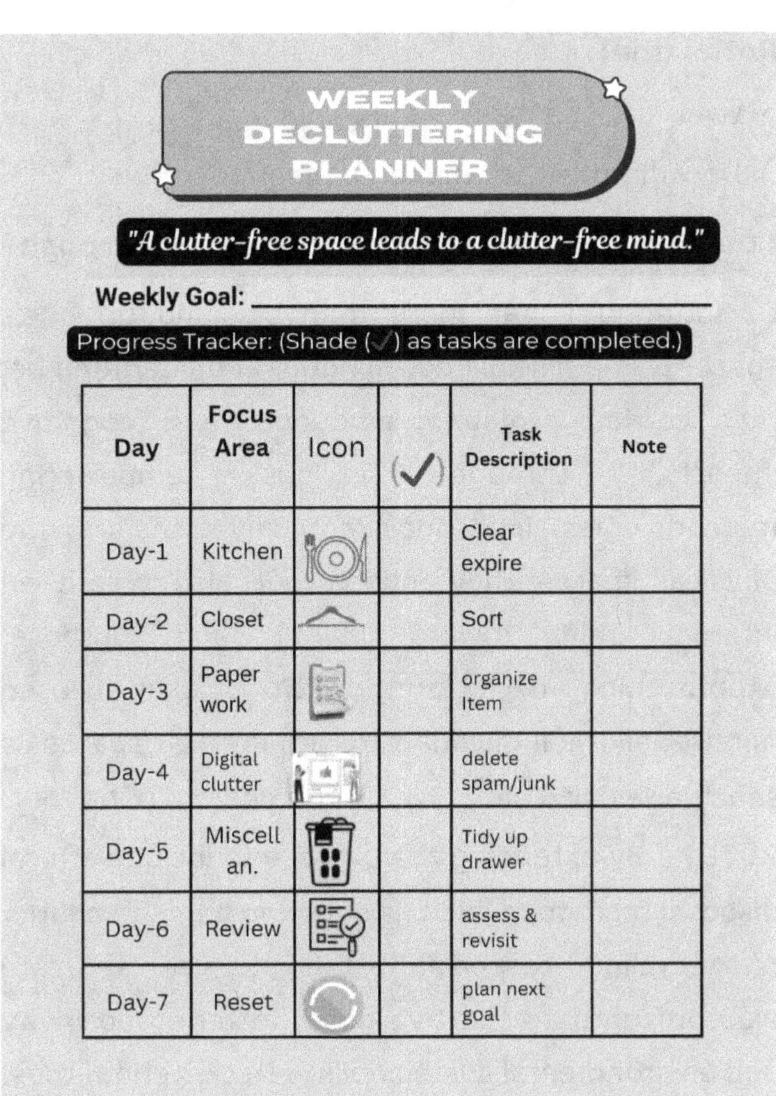

Day	Focus Area	Icon	(✓)	Task Description	Note
Day-1	Kitchen			Clear expire	
Day-2	Closet			Sort	
Day-3	Paper work			organize Item	
Day-4	Digital clutter			delete spam/junk	
Day-5	Miscell an.			Tidy up drawer	
Day-6	Review			assess & revisit	
Day-7	Reset			plan next goal	

Figure 6. Weekly decluttering planner by item and action

Reflection:

1) What worked well? What could improve?
2) How did this task make you feel?

Conclusion: Cultivating a Lifestyle of Purpose

Decluttering is far more than cleaning up one's space. It is a disciplined, mindful, and liberating act that carries profound emotional and cognitive impacts. Through various empowering methodologies, individuals not only transform the physical spaces they inhabit but also create an internal shift toward clarity and purpose. "Approaching decluttering with a gain-focused mindset allows individuals to reclaim their spaces as sanctuaries of calm, joy, and freedom (Chatzky, 2019)." By extending the practice to include ethical disposal methods—such as donating items to charity or recycling responsibly—this act of self-care blossoms into a collective good, fostering positivity and environmental sustainability. Decluttering, thus, is a pathway to serenity and meaning in an increasingly chaotic world.

Chapter 5: Living with Less

Embracing the Principles of Minimalism

In today's world, where consumerism often equates happiness with acquiring more, the philosophy of minimalism emerges as a countercultural yet deeply meaningful approach to life. Minimalism isn't about deprivation; instead, it's about intentionally choosing simplicity to focus on what truly matters. The art of living with less isn't about the number of items you own; it's about fostering a mindful relationship with your possessions and prioritizing quality, purpose, and gratitude. This chapter focuses on the core principles of minimalism, guiding you to uncover your "enough," adopt a quality-over-quantity mindset, and embrace gratitude as a transformative practice for intentional living.

Defining Your "Enough"

Minimalism begins with understanding what "enough" means for you personally. This process is deeply introspective—a journey of differentiating your true needs from your wants. It's about stripping away external pressures to uncover the essentials that align with your values and lifestyle.

How to Define Your Enough

Ask Reflective Questions: Start by asking yourself: Which items do I truly need to feel comfortable and functional in my daily life? What possessions bring genuine joy or add meaningful value to my existence? Which things could I release without a sense of loss?

Focus on Function and Purpose: Pinpoint what enables you to live contentedly without excess. Evaluate whether an item serves its purpose well or simply takes up space.

Personalizing Your Minimalism

Your definition of enough is entirely unique. By answering these questions, you create a framework for making decisions about which belongings to retain and which to let go. From this clarity, you can build a lifestyle truly aligned with your needs—free of unnecessary clutter but enriched with meaningful possessions.

Creating an Inventory of Essentials

Once you understand your definition of "enough," the next step is to assess your current belongings and create a personal inventory. This practice not only declutters your life but also reinforces a conscious simplicity by categorizing your possessions.

Steps to Build Your Inventory:

List Your Essentials: Identify the items you rely on daily or weekly. These might include pieces of clothing, kitchen tools, or gadgets. Highlight their importance and usefulness in your routine.

Evaluate Sentimental Items: Recognize belongings tied to memories. Keep only those that evoke joy or hold significant meaning to your personal story. Let go of items lying idle that no longer resonate.

Identify What Can Be Released: Dive into the cornered clutter—possessions collecting dust. Decide whether to donate, recycle, or discard these items with thoughtfulness.

Benefits of a Personal Inventory

This reflective inventory process helps streamline your environment, ensuring that everything remaining has a purpose or value. Over time, this practice reduces the emotional and mental weight of excess, leaving you with a space that breathes simplicity and intent.

The Value of Quality Over Quantity

A cornerstone of minimalism is shifting focus from amassing numerous possessions to choosing high-quality, versatile ones. This approach not only reduces clutter but also ensures that every item serves a meaningful purpose.

How to Prioritize Quality

Durability First: Choose items made from materials designed to last—sturdy clothing, reliable kitchen tools, or long-lasting furniture. High-quality products reduce the need for frequent replacements, saving resources and reducing waste.

Versatility Matters: Select multipurpose items wherever possible. For example, a cast iron skillet can be used for various cooking techniques, while modular furniture adapts to changing needs.

Mindful Purchasing: Before any purchase, ask yourself: Will this item genuinely enhance my life? Does it align with the lifestyle I'm curating? This question helps avoid impulsive buying and ensures new additions hold significance.

Benefits of Choosing Quality

Focusing on quality drives conscious consumption and promotes long-term satisfaction. Your living spaces become more streamlined, functional, and aesthetically pleasing, reinforcing the essence of a life lived with intention.

Cultivating a Gratitude Practice

Gratitude is a transformative component of minimalism. By appreciating what you already have, the desire for excess diminishes, leaving space for contentment and simplicity to thrive.

Techniques to Foster Gratitude:

Daily Reflections: Spend just a few minutes each day reflecting on the things you're grateful for. It could be simple pleasures like a warm cup of tea, a favorite book, or the support of loved ones.

Gratitude Journaling: Maintain a journal and write down three things you appreciate each day. This consistent practice helps center your attention on abundance rather than what's missing.

Mindful Consumption: Before purchasing something new, pause and ask, "Do I truly need this? Will it add value to my life?" Reflecting on these questions encourages thoughtful choices.

Expressing Appreciation: Share your gratitude with others. A simple "thank you" or an act of kindness can deepen relationships and promote a culture of appreciation.

Why Gratitude Matters

Gratitude shifts focus from lack to abundance, transforming how you view your life and possessions. As part of your minimalist journey, it fosters a sense of fulfillment, making the pursuit of more feel unnecessary while enhancing the joy found in what you already have.

Conclusion

Minimalism is not just about owning fewer things; it's a lifestyle of embracing what truly matters. By defining your "enough," creating an inventory of essentials, focusing on quality over quantity, and practicing gratitude, you can transform your life in meaningful ways.

Each step you take toward minimalism creates space—both physical and mental—for what brings you joy and fulfillment. The weight of unnecessary possessions lifts, making room for freedom, clarity, and enriched living. Through this intentional approach, you'll discover the profound beauty of simplicity—where having less allows you to experience more.

As you embark on this journey, remember that minimalism is deeply personal. It's not a rigid set of rules but a path to curating a life that aligns with your values. Embrace the liberation, the calm, and the sense of purpose that comes with living intentionally.

Chapter 6: Consumer-Conscious Lifestyle

In an era where consumerism is often celebrated, it becomes increasingly necessary to cultivate a lifestyle conscious of consumption. This chapter delves into several practical strategies to help individuals establish spending boundaries, detox from social media and advertisements, and prioritize experiences over tangible possessions. Adhering to these principles can foster a more balanced and meaningful existence, aligning financial practices with personal values.

Setting Spending Boundaries

The first step toward a consumer-conscious lifestyle is establishing clear spending boundaries. A well-structured monthly budget is a critical tool in this pursuit, providing a framework for tracking income and expenses effectively.

Create a Monthly Budget: To construct a robust budget, one should start with a comprehensive understanding of income sources, including salary, freelance work, and other streams of revenue.

Subsequently, categorize expenses into fixed costs, such as rent and utilities, and variable costs, like groceries and leisure activities. After listing these expenses, it is essential to set realistic limits for each category that not only account for immediate needs but also incorporate savings goals. At the end of each month, a thorough review of expenditures against the established budget will identify areas for potential improvement, reinforcing informed financial choices aligned with one's aspirations.

Implement a "One-In, One-Out" Rule: To counteract the compulsive nature of material accumulation, the "one-in, one-out" rule proves invaluable. "Implementing a 'one-in, one-out' rule helps counteract compulsive material accumulation (Becker, 2016)." This principle advocates for mindfulness in consumption, compelling individuals to relinquish an existing item for every new purchase made. Before indulging in shopping activities, one should identify a specific item that can be part of a decluttering process. Scheduling regular decluttering sessions aids in recognizing items that no longer serve a purpose or elicit joy. Once identified, these items can be donated or sold, thereby supporting others and affirming a commitment to a simplified lifestyle. This approach ultimately facilitates a balanced relationship with material possessions, reducing physical and mental clutter.

Detoxing from Social Media and Advertisements

The pressure of consumerism is greatly amplified by the pervasive nature of social media. To cultivate a more conscious consumer mindset, it is crucial to detox from these influences and approach online interactions with intent.

Unfollow Accounts That Promote Consumerism: Engaging in an audit of one's social media feeds is a critical step in this detoxification process. By unfollowing accounts that propagate excessive consumerism or trigger feelings of inadequacy regarding personal possessions, one can significantly improve their online experience. Instead, seek out influencers who promote minimalism, sustainability, and mindful living. Curating content tailored to personal values enables individuals to focus on the aspects of life that truly matter.

Use Ad Blockers and Avoid Impulse-Prone Platforms: The barrage of advertisements is often a catalyst for impulsive purchasing behaviors. Installing ad-blocking software can reduce exposure to targeted ads while browsing online, mitigating the temptation to purchase spontaneously. Moreover, during major sales events, it is prudent to pre-determine purchases rather than succumbing to the allure of discounts. Practicing mindful browsing—being selective about the platforms engaged with—can further enhance the consumer-conscious lifestyle, freeing individuals from the pressure exerted by consumer-driven environments.

Emphasizing Experiences Over Material Things

One of the most profound methodologies for fostering a consumer-conscious lifestyle involves redirecting financial resources toward experiences rather than accumulating material possessions. Research consistently indicates that experiences contribute more significantly to long-term happiness than do physical items.

"Redirecting spending toward meaningful experiences—such as travel, personal development courses, and shared activities with loved ones—creates lasting memories and enhances overall well-being (Csikszentmihalyi, 1990)." By valuing life's moments over material acquisitions, individuals not only cultivate deeper connections with themselves and others but also redefine their relationship with consumption. This shift in perspective fosters a more enriching and fulfilling lifestyle.

In conclusion, cultivating a consumer-conscious lifestyle necessitates intentional actions across various facets of personal finance and social interactions. By establishing spending boundaries, detoxing from pervasive consumer influences, and prioritizing experiences over possessions, individuals can forge a path towards a balanced existence that honors both their values and well-being.

Creating a consumer-conscious lifestyle requires a deliberate shift in perspective, particularly in a world where advertisements and media constantly encourage us to buy more. The essence of this lifestyle is finding balance between needs, values, and consumption while avoiding the trap of overindulgence. Through practical and purposeful measures, one can take steps to control spending, willingly part with unnecessary objects, detach from advertisement-driven platforms, and cherish the value of experiences over material goods.

Setting Spending Boundaries

One of the foundational elements of a consumer-conscious lifestyle is establishing spending boundaries. This entails aligning financial behaviors with both personal priorities and broader life goals. To successfully achieve this, a methodical, disciplined approach to budgeting is crucial.

Creating a Monthly Budget

A monthly budget permits an individual to systematically allocate income while tailoring spending to specific priorities. Follow these steps to build an effective budget:

Track Your Income: Start by recording every source of income, no matter how small. This includes your salary, part-time engagements, freelancer payments, and any other revenue streams. A comprehensive view of your earnings helps build clarity on what is available for allocation.

Categorize Your Expenses: Break down your monthly expenses into categories like fixed costs (e.g., mortgage/rent, utilities, insurance) and variable expenses (e.g., dining out, entertainment, groceries). Understanding where each dollar is going is key to identifying unnecessary expenditures.

Set Realistic Limits: For each category, allocate specific spending limits. These limits should be achievable without neglecting necessary savings. For instance, instead of budgeting excessively for luxuries, direct more funds toward investment or emergency reserves.

Review and Adjust Regularly: Make it a habit at the end of each month to compare actual spending against the pre-set budget. Look for patterns of overspending and adjust the next month's budget accordingly. This feedback loop ensures continuous improvement in money management.

By following these steps, a carefully constructed budget becomes not only a tool for financial management but a means for an individual to align their material life closely with their values and aspirations.

Implementing the "One-In, One-Out" Rule

Accumulating unnecessary objects often leads to physical clutter and mental unrest. "By adopting the one-in, one-out approach, individuals can maintain a more mindful and intentional relationship with their possessions (Becker, 2016)." This simple yet effective practice ensures that each acquisition is balanced by letting go of something already owned.

Before Shopping, Reflect and Plan: Before making a purchase, think carefully about its necessity and purpose. Identify an item you are willing to part with as a trade-off. This encourages mindfulness and avoids spur-of-the-moment buying behavior.

Conduct Regular Decluttering Sessions: Set aside specific times to review your belongings. Focus on items no longer used, no longer fitting your needs, or failing to bring joy. Regular decluttering sessions become a therapeutic activity, allowing you to assess the true value of what you own.

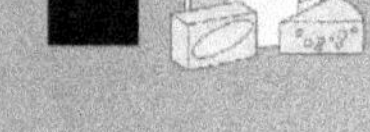
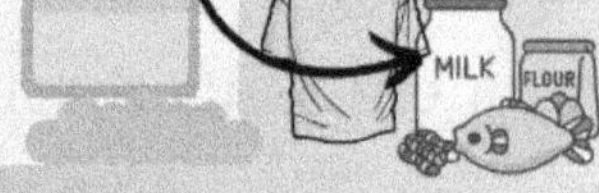

"Simplify YourSpace with the - One in -One Out Rule"

"For every new item brought into your home, one existing item must leave."

"Declutter Your Home, Simplify Your Life."

Decluttering Benefits:
Less clutter
Helping others
Financial savings
Joyful living

Decluttering steps:
Step 1: Identify a new item before shopping.
Step 2: Choose one item to declutter.
Step 3: Decide to donate, sell, or recycle.
Step 4: Schedule regular decluttering sessions.

Decluttering check list:
Does it serve a purpose?
Does it spark joy?
Has it been used in the last year?
Is it worth keeping over something new?

MILK
FLOUR

Figure 7. Illustration showing "decluttering your life inspired by the idea with the one in-one out rule (Becker, 2016)."

Donate or Sell Items: Instead of simply discarding what you no longer need, consider donating items to those who can make use of them or selling them in online platforms and second-hand markets. Not only does this contribute to sustainability, but it also reinforces the habit of mindful living.

By maintaining the "one-in, one-out" principle, one slowly reduces their consumption footprint while cultivating a deliberate approach to ownership. It's a proactive way to take charge of material possessions and restore harmony in living spaces.

Detoxing from Social Media and Advertisements

The influence of modern media in shaping consumer behaviors is unparalleled. Social media advertisements, celebrity endorsements, and even curated lifestyles on platforms often promote unattainable standards of wealth and happiness, feeding compulsive consumption. Detoxifying digital spaces is imperative for nurturing a consumer-conscious mindset.

Unfollow Accounts That Promote Consumerism

Social media accounts often glamorize excessive consumerism by showcasing abundant possessions or luxurious lifestyles. Detox your feed by taking these actions:

Audit Your Social Media Feed: Regularly evaluate the accounts you follow. Unfollow pages that promote excessive materialism or perpetuate feelings of inadequacy.

Follow Positive Role Models: Seek out influencers known for their focus on sustainability, minimalism, or mindful living. Such role models encourage a shift in mentality towards valuing simplicity and experiences.

Curate Your Online Space: Use social media tools cautiously by enhancing your feeds with interests that resonate with personal values, such as wellness, education, or creativity. By personalizing your experience, you can let go of the relentless consumerist narrative.

Using Ad Blockers and Practicing Mindful Engagement

Advertisements hijack consumer priorities by creating a perpetual state of urgency or desire for products. Taking countermeasures to block or avoid impulsive shopping avenues can help regain control over purchasing decisions.

Install Efficient Ad Blockers: Ad-blocking applications can eliminate intrusive advertisements while browsing online, keeping distractions to a minimum.

Avoid Shopping Platforms During Sales Peaks: Whether it's Black Friday or seasonal clearances, major sales events often lead to unplanned purchasing. Plan ahead for items you truly need and steer clear of impulse-driven platforms.

Take Breaks from Shopping Sites: Being mindful of the websites and apps you interact with is vital. If possible, reduce engagement with platforms that foster consumerism and redirect the time saved into other fulfilling activities.

Integrating ad blockers and practicing strategic browsing fosters intentional purchasing habits and helps individuals develop a healthier perspective on what they really need versus momentary desires.

Emphasizing Experiences Over Material Things

Turning your attention away from accumulating possessions and embracing meaningful experiences offers a profound way to enhance life satisfaction. Numerous studies have indicated that experiences bring people closer, provide long-lasting fulfillment, and engrain deeper emotional attachment compared to physical items.

Invest in Experiences Worth Remembering

Redirect funds typically allocated for material indulgences toward cherished experiences that create lasting memories. Here's how:

Prioritize Activities with Loved Ones: Whether it's a family vacation, a shared dinner, or a fun workshop, such activities strengthen relationships and foster togetherness.

Seek Personal Growth: Invest in education, mentorship programs, or skill-building courses that contribute to long-term personal development and satisfaction.

Focus on Quality Time: Reduce superfluous shopping activities and channel that time into pursuits like hiking, visiting art exhibitions, or trying new hobbies.

By valuing experiences, individuals not only cultivate happiness that extends beyond the instant gratification of a purchase but also discover meaning in simplicity, connection, and personal enrichment.

Conclusion

By integrating thoughtful measures like setting spending boundaries, adhering to decluttering principles, detoxing from social media, and prioritizing experiences over material things, cultivating a consumer-conscious lifestyle becomes achievable. The journey towards this lifestyle is one of reclaiming control, reducing stressors, and realigning financial habits with deeply held values. Far from being an exercise in deprivation, it's an invitation to embrace a more meaningful existence— one where life's richest experiences take precedence over transient possessions and superficial contentment. Meaningful living begins not with endless accumulation but with deliberate and purposeful choices. The ebbs and flows of such a path ultimately yield heightened mindfulness and life satisfaction.

Chapter 7: Building Sustainable Habits

Creating sustainable habits is essential for maintaining a lifestyle rooted in minimalism and intentional living. For instance, "setting up a designated space free of clutter can create a sense of calm and focus (Becker, 2016) ". Regularly reflecting on whether possessions add value can help prevent overconsumption; for example, identifying items unused for months may reveal opportunities to simplify. Additionally, teaching children to appreciate quality over quantity, such as encouraging them to choose a single cherished toy over multiple fleeting purchases, instills the principles of mindful consumption in the next generation.

Create Intentional Environment

An intentional environment is a consciously designed space that fosters simplicity and clarity, allowing individuals to prioritize what truly matters. Simplicity streamlines distractions and reduces clutter, while clarity provides focus and direction, making it easier to identify and act on core values. For instance, an office free from unnecessary items and interruptions can help an individual remain focused on completing meaningful tasks, ensuring that time and energy are devoted to what truly matters. To achieve this, several strategies can be employed:

Declutter Regularly: Begin by removing items that no longer serve a purpose or bring joy. Tools such as donation bins or decluttering apps can facilitate this process, transforming it into a liberating experience that enhances the serenity of one's space.

Designate Spaces: Organizing the home into specific areas for distinct activities—such as a reading nook, workspace, or relaxation zone—enhances functionality and encourages mindful engagement in these activities.

Use Minimalist Decor: Opt for simple yet meaningful decor. Selecting a few key pieces that resonate personally rather than overwhelming the space with numerous items contributes to a cleaner environment.

Incorporate Natural Elements: Introducing plants or natural materials can foster a sense of calm and connection to nature, enriching the overall ambiance of the home.

Maintain Clutter-Free Zones

Establishing and maintaining clutter-free zones are critical for cultivating an intentional environment, as they promote mental clarity and focus by reducing distractions. To achieve this:

Choose Key Areas: Identify specific locations in the home, such as entryways or dining tables, that will remain clutter-free.

Set Rules: Implement guidelines for these zones, such as prohibiting items left on surfaces or limiting decorative pieces, to promote mindfulness regarding what enters these spaces.

Regular Maintenance: Schedule weekly tidying sessions to prevent clutter accumulation. A few minutes of upkeep can maintain clarity and organization.

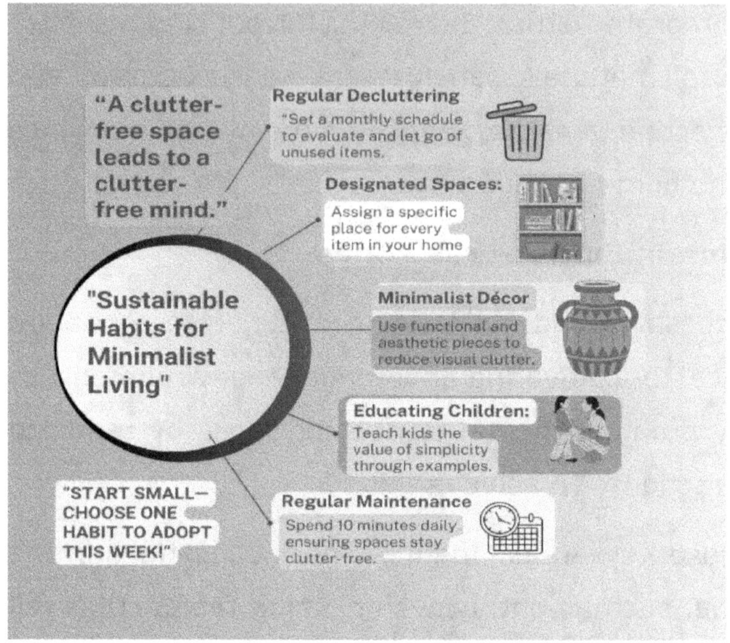

Figure 8. illustration on Sustainable habits of minimalist lifestyle by adopting different strategies.

Check-In Regularly

Regular assessments are vital for sustaining a minimalist lifestyle. Scheduling biannual decluttering sessions can help individuals reassess their belongings and ensure alignment with personal values:

Set a Calendar Reminder: Designate specific dates, such as the beginning of spring and fall, for decluttering sessions to establish a routine.

Involve Family Members: Encourage participation from family members to foster a collective commitment to minimalism.

Review Each Category: Tackle one category at a time—such as clothing, kitchenware, or books—during each session to make the process manageable.

Decide on Disposition: For each item, reflect on whether it adds value or joy to life. If it does not, consider donating, recycling, or discarding it.

Reflect on What Truly Adds Value

During decluttering, it is crucial to reflect on which items genuinely enhance one's life. Techniques to facilitate this reflection include:

Journaling: Maintain a journal to document insights gained after each decluttering session, focusing on consumption habits and personal values.

Mindfulness Practice: Incorporate mindfulness techniques during reflections, meditating on gratitude for valuable items while acknowledging those that no longer serve a purpose.

Adjust Goals: Use insights from reflections to adjust future purchasing goals, ensuring they align with values and positively contribute to life.

Teach the Next Generation

Instilling mindful habits in children and family members is essential for fostering a sustainable lifestyle across generations. This practice not only benefits individuals but also has a positive ripple effect, enhancing family dynamics and contributing to a more responsible and conscious society over time. This can be achieved by:

Leading by Example: Demonstrating minimalism in daily life serves as a powerful teaching tool, encouraging family members to adopt similar habits.

In conclusion, building sustainable habits for intentional living requires a committed approach to creating an intentional environment, regular self-assessment, and the education of future generations.

Chapter8: Minimalism Rewards

Emotional and Psychological Benefits

Embracing a minimalist lifestyle and fostering a clutter-free environment can yield profound emotional and psychological benefits. This chapter explores how minimalism reduces stress, enhances productivity, liberates individuals from consumer-driven comparison traps, and fosters a renewed sense of purpose. Discover how living with less creates space for more—more joy, clarity, and meaning.

Reduced Stress and Increased Productivity

The Connection Between Clutter, Stress, and Mental Clarity

Clutter overwhelms the senses, elevates stress, and diminishes productivity. Studies reveal that disorder disrupts focus and hinders decision-making. In contrast, "a minimalist environment provides a sanctuary of clarity and calm (Chatzky, 2019)."

Enhanced Focus: A tidy space minimizes distractions, enabling sharper concentration and efficient problem-solving.

Mental Clarity: Fewer visual and mental distractions enhance creativity and decision-making.

Lower Stress Levels: Organized surroundings reduce cortisol, the stress hormone, fostering a serene atmosphere.

Increased Productivity: An environment that supports your goals boosts confidence and motivation.

"Why Minimalism Matters"

Benefit	Description
Reduced Stress	Fosters a serene and calming environment.
Enhanced Productivity	Promotes focus and task efficiency.
Boosted Self-Worth	Shifts focus from comparison to personal contentment.
Clarity of Purpose	Aligns daily choices with core values.
Deeper Relationships	Prioritizes meaningful connections over possessions.

Infographic: Key Benefits of Minimalism

Figure 9: Shows the different benefits of minimalism for stress reduction and enhance productivity

Actionable Steps to Create a Clutter-Free Environment

- Start Small: Begin with one drawer or shelf to avoid overwhelm.
- One-In-One-Out Rule: Remove an old item for every new one acquired.
- Prioritize Essentials: Keep only items with clear purpose or genuine joy.
- Decluttering Schedule: Dedicate regular time to organization.
- Purpose-Focused Zones: Designate areas for work, relaxation, and creativity.

Freedom from the Comparison Trap

Escaping the Chains of Consumerism

Modern society often equates material wealth with success, trapping individuals in endless comparisons. Minimalism shifts the focus from external validation to internal contentment.

Redefining Success: Minimalism emphasizes fulfillment through experiences and growth over accumulation.

Increased Self-Worth: Letting go of comparisons fosters confidence and a healthier self-image.

Contentment with Simplicity: Gratitude for what you have replaces longing for what you lack.

Stronger Relationships: Prioritizing people over possessions strengthens connections.

Practical Strategies to Break Free from Consumerism

1. Audit Social Media

Message:

"Take control of your social media experience by following accounts that inspire positivity and align with your values. Remember, social media is a tool—curate it to uplift and motivate, not to compare and despair."

Actions:

Review Your Feed:

Spend 30 minutes scrolling through your social media feeds and note accounts that spark envy or negative emotions.

Unfollow or mute these accounts.

Curate Positivity:

Follow accounts that promote minimalism, self-care, mindfulness, or whatever aligns with your goals.

Examples include thought leaders, motivational speakers, or communities centered on wellness and intentional living.

Limit Exposure:

Set screen time limits to avoid endless scrolling that fosters unhealthy comparisons.

2. Practice Gratitude

Message:

"Gratitude shifts your perspective from lack to abundance. Begin and end your day by reflecting on the things you're grateful for—it's a small step that fosters lasting happiness."

Actions:

Start a Gratitude Journal:

Dedicate a notebook or app to record three things you're grateful for each day.

Example entries: A sunny day, a supportive friend, or a productive work session.

Express Gratitude to Others:

Send thank-you messages or verbal expressions of appreciation to people who positively impact your life.

Example: "Thank you for helping me through my project. Your support means a lot."

Practice Gratitude Meditation:

Dedicate 5–10 minutes to reflect on the blessings in your life. Apps like Calm or Headspace can help guide you.

3. Invest in Experiences

Message:

"Objects fade, but memories last forever. Prioritize experiences that bring joy and connection—they enrich your life in ways possessions never can."

Actions:

Plan Experience-Oriented Activities:

Research local or virtual events like community workshops, outdoor hikes, or art classes.

Block time in your calendar to ensure these experiences are prioritized.

Shift Gift-Giving Habits:

Replace physical gifts with experiential ones, like tickets to a concert, a cooking class, or a trip.

Example: Instead of buying clothes for a friend, organize a day out together.

Capture Moments Creatively:

- Start a photo diary or create scrapbooks to document meaningful experiences.
- This practice helps you relive the joy and reinforces the value of those memories.

4. Set Personal Goals

Message:

"Define success on your terms. By setting goals aligned with your values, you pave the way for meaningful progress and fulfillment."

Actions:

Write Down SMART Goals:

Create goals that are Specific, Measurable, Achievable, Relevant, and Time-bound.

Example: "I will read one book on personal growth each month for the next three months."

Break Goals into Steps:

Divide large goals into actionable tasks.

Example: For a fitness goal, list tasks like "Sign up for a gym," "Buy workout clothes," and "Create a weekly workout schedule."

Track Progress Regularly:

- Use a planner, app, or habit tracker to measure achievements.
- Celebrate milestones, even small ones, to maintain motivation.

5. Mindful Shopping

Message:

"Before you buy, pause and reflect. Does this item bring true joy or serve a real purpose? Thoughtful purchases make life lighter and more meaningful."

Actions:

Adopt the 24-Hour Rule:

Delay non-essential purchases for 24 hours. This cooling-off period helps assess whether you truly need or want the item.

Example: Instead of impulse-buying a gadget, sleep on it and revisit the decision.

Create a Shopping List:

- Write down items you need before going shopping, and stick to it.
- This practice reduces impulsive buys and keeps you focused on essentials.

Embrace Minimalism:

For every new item you buy, donate or discard an old one.

Example: If you buy a new sweater, remove one you no longer wear.

Each strategy involves actionable steps paired with a motivational message that reinforces the value of minimalism and helps individuals resist consumerism effectively.

A New Sense of Purpose

Living Intentionally and Aligned with Your Values

Minimalism isn't just decluttering—it's a mindset promoting intentional living. Removing distractions allows alignment with core values.

- o *Clarity of Purpose:* Identify what brings true fulfillment.
- o *Intentional Choices:* Spend time and resources meaningfully.
- o *Empowerment Through Simplicity:* Focusing on essentials energizes passions and goals.
- o *Community Connection:* Simplifying creates space to contribute time and resources to others.

Steps to Define and Live by Your Values

- o Reflect on Priorities: Identify activities and relationships that bring joy.
- o Document Core Values: Write guiding principles for meaningful living.
- o Evaluate Habits: Ensure routines align with values.

o   Set Aligned Goals: Dedicate effort to value-driven activities.

o   Revisit and Adjust: Periodically review to maintain harmony.

Overcoming Obstacles to a Clutter-Free Lifestyle

Challenges like emotional attachments, busy schedules, and societal pressures can impede minimalism. Overcome these with practical strategies:

- *Emotional Attachments*: Keep items that genuinely reflect cherished memories.
- *Time Constraints:* Dedicate short, consistent intervals to decluttering.
- *Lack of Systems:* Establish organizational methods for long-term order.
- *Consumer Culture Pressures*: Remind yourself of minimalism's core values.
- *Procrastination:* Break tasks into manageable steps and celebrate progress.

Conclusion: From Chaos to Clarity

As we conclude this transformative journey from overconsumption to intentional living, it's essential to celebrate the progress you've made. Embracing minimalism and creating a clutter-free environment is not just about physical space; it's a profound shift in mindset that fosters a life filled with purpose and fulfillment. By prioritizing what truly matters, you have taken significant steps toward enhancing your emotional and psychological well-being.

The Impact of Decluttering on Emotional Well-Being

Decluttering your physical space has a direct influence on your emotional health. A clean and organized environment reduces stress and anxiety, allowing for greater mental clarity and focus. Studies show that clutter can overwhelm our senses, leading to feelings of chaos that mirror our internal state. By removing excess items, you create a serene atmosphere that promotes relaxation and calmness, making your home a sanctuary rather than a source of stress. This sense of control over your environment not only boosts your mood but also enhances your self-esteem, as you experience the satisfaction of achieving a more organized life.

Common Misconceptions About Decluttering and Minimalism

While the benefits of decluttering are clear, several misconceptions can hinder progress. One common myth is that minimalism means living with as few possessions as possible, which can feel daunting or unrealistic. In reality, minimalism is about making intentional choices that align with your values—keeping what brings you joy and letting go of what doesn't. Another misconception is that decluttering is a one-time effort; in truth, it's an ongoing practice that requires regular maintenance and reflection. Recognizing these misconceptions allows you to approach minimalism with a mindset focused on personal growth rather than strict limitations.

Encouraging Ongoing Mindfulness

As you continue on this path toward intentional living, remember that mindfulness is key to maintaining the progress you've achieved. Regularly check in with yourself—reflect on what adds value to your life and what may need reevaluation. Embrace the practice of gratitude, celebrating the simple joys that come from living with less.

Incorporate routines that support your commitment to minimalism, whether through biannual decluttering sessions or daily habits that promote organization. Surround yourself with supportive communities or resources that inspire you to stay true to your values.

Ultimately, the journey from chaos to clarity is ongoing. Embrace each step along the way as an opportunity for growth and discovery. As you cultivate a lifestyle of intentionality, you'll find that clarity not only transforms your physical space but also enriches every aspect of your life.

Thank you for embarking on this journey toward minimalism and intentional livig. May your path be filled with peace, purpose, and profound joy as you continue to embrace the beauty of simplicity.

Glossary

- **Consumerism**: "The belief that personal happiness depends on purchasing material **Consumerism: "The belief that personal happiness depends on purchasing material possessions (Kasser, 2002)."**

- **Minimalism:** "A lifestyle choice focused on living with only what is necessary (Kondo, 2014)."

- **Decluttering:** "The process of removing unneeded or excess items from your space (Becker, 2016)."

- **Consumer-Conscious:** "A mindset focused on mindful and intentional consumption, avoiding impulsive or excessive spending (Becker, 2016)."

- **Mental Clarity:** "A state of focused and clear thinking, often achieved by

reducing distractions and clutter
(Chatzky, 2019)."

- **Mindful Shopping:** "The practice of making deliberate purchasing decisions that align with values and long-term goals (Kondo, 2014)."

- **Spending Boundaries:** "Limits set on financial expenditures to prioritize needs, save, and avoid debt (Smith, 2019)."

- **Possessions:** "Items owned by an individual, often categorized as essential, sentimental, or unnecessary (Becker, 2016)."

References

1. Kasser, T. (2002). *The High Price of Materialism*. Cambridge: MIT Press.

2. Brown, B. (2012). *Daring Greatly: How the Courage to Be Vulnerable Transforms the Way We Live, Love, Parent, and Lead*. Gotham Books.

3. Kondo, M. (2014). *The Life-Changing Magic of Tidying Up: The Japanese Art of Decluttering and Organizing*. Ten Speed Press.

4. Csikszentmihalyi, M. (1990). *Flow: The Psychology of Optimal Experience*. Harper & Row.

5. Smith, A. (2019). "The Psychology of Decluttering: Why Letting Go Feels Good." *Journal of Consumer Psychology*, 25(3), 145-159.

6. Chatzky, J. (2019). "How Clutter Impacts Your Financial and Mental Health." *Forbes Magazine*.

7. Becker, J. (2016). *The More of Less: Finding the Life You Want Under Everything You Own*. WaterBrook Press.

8. Carver, C. (2017). *Soulful Simplicity: How Living with Less Can Lead to So Much More*. Penguin Random House.

9. McKeown, G. (2021). *Effortless: Make It Easier to Do What Matters Most*. Currency.

Additional Resources

Websites on Minimalism and Mindful Living:

1. *Becoming Minimalist*

   (https://www.becomingminimalist.com)

   o Features articles and tips on living with less and finding purpose.

2. *The Minimalists*

   (https://www.theminimalists.com)

   o Provides podcasts, blog posts, and community resources for simplifying life.

3. *Mindful.org* (https://www.mindful.org)

   o A platform dedicated to mindfulness practices and intentional living.

Apps for Spending and Decluttering:

1. **Mint** (https://mint.intuit.com)

   o A budgeting app that helps track spending habits.

2. **YNAB (You Need A Budget)**

   (https://www.youneedabudget.com)

- o Offers financial planning tools to reduce unnecessary expenses.

3. **Sortly** (https://www.sortly.com)

   - o An inventory and decluttering app to help organize personal belongings.

4. **Declutter** (https://www.decluttr.com)

   - o A platform for selling unwanted items.

Online Tools and Blogs for Further Learning:

1. *TED Talks:*

   - o "Less Stuff, More Happiness" by Graham Hill (https://www.ted.com).

2. *Medium Articles:*

   - o Topics on decluttering, mindfulness, and sustainable living.

3. *Simplicity Collective* (https://www.simplicitycollective.com)

   - o Focused on simple living and sustainability.

About the Author

Yimam Beshir is a seasoned public health professional with over 15 years of experience dedicated to enhancing community health through education, advocacy, and evidence-based practices. With a Master's degree in Public Health, Yimam has made significant contributions across diverse public health domains, including environmental health, wellness, and sanitation.

Driven by a passion for personal growth and sustainable living, Yimam emphasizes the importance of fostering a healthy lifestyle while protecting the environment. His work highlights critical issues such as resource conservation, safe material disposal, and the prevention of ecological harm caused by waste and overconsumption. Yimam advocates for conscious practices like minimalism and decluttering as tools for achieving a balanced life and preserving the planet.

This dedication inspired him to author *Declutter Your Life for Peace and Purpose: A Practical Guide to Mindful Living and Simplified Spaces*. In this book, Yimam blends his academic expertise with actionable insights, offering readers practical strategies to cultivate holistic wellness and personal development.

Beyond his professional endeavors, Yimam is deeply committed to community service and mentoring the next generation of public health professionals. His unwavering dedication to lifelong learning and helping others embodies his mission to create a healthier, more sustainable future for all.

Call to Action

Thank you for taking the time to embark on this journey with me. Your support means the world, and I am truly grateful that you've allowed my work to be a part of your life.

If you enjoyed this book, I would greatly appreciate it if you could leave a review on Amazon. Your feedback not only helps me improve but also helps other readers discover this work. Every review makes a difference!

I'd love to stay connected with you. Join my email list for exclusive updates, practical tips, and early access to upcoming projects. You can also follow me on social media, where I share insights, inspiration, and behind-the-scenes glimpses into my creative process.

Email signup: https://sites.google.com/view/tosa-online-bussiness/signup-form

Twitter: http://twitter.com/@Yimam00669351

YouTube: https://www.youtube.com/@Tossa-Health-Wealth

Acknowledgment of Reader's Efforts

To you, the reader—thank you for investing your time and energy into this book. Your curiosity, commitment, and willingness to explore new ideas are what make this journey worthwhile. You've taken an important step by diving into these pages, and I hope they've inspired you, challenged your perspective, and added value to your life.

Now, take that next step! Share your thoughts, connect with me, and let's continue this journey together. Your voice matters, and your story is just as important as the one you've read here. Thank you for being.